Adrenal Fatigue Diet Cookbook

Table of Content

Introduction

Our body works in mysterious ways, it is not only adaptive to external changes but also mimics those through the functioning of its organs and related hormones. This is the reason that it quickly becomes the manifestation of what we eat and what we do. Our every busy lifestyle has made us more ignorant towards the body needs and more obsessed with work and work. And for this reason, many symptoms emerge which are not even the part of any medical diagnosis yet. Adrenal fatigue is also such condition which is apparently caused by 'chronic stresses and 'adrenal inefficiency.' After minutely observing all the symptoms and complication related to this condition, experts have come down to one most effective resolution, and that is Adrenal Fatigue diet. From the basics of the condition to the complete list of recipes, this book is designed to provide an essential guide to those who are suffering from its symptoms.

What is Adrenal Fatigue?

The word Adrenal comes from the 'Adrenal Glands' which are present on human Kidneys. These glands are responsible for producing hormones named 'Cortisol' which help in maintaining the blood pressure in 'stressful' situations. With chronic stress or inefficiency of the adrenal glands, enough cortisol is not released which can cause low blood pressure. Adrenal hormones are also responsible for various other bodily functions and aid the execution of those processes. Therefore adrenal inefficiency is also directly or indirectly linked to various other symptoms. These include:

- Body pain
- Digestive problems
- Weight loss
- Loss of appetite
- Nervousness

- Body fatigue
- Low blood pressure
- Lightheadedness
- Stomach pain
- Muscle weakness
- The weakness of the immune system.

In severe cases, constant adrenal fatigue can cause:

- hyperpigmentation
- nausea
- depression
- diarrhea
- vomiting

Adrenal Fatigue Diet:

Conditions like adrenal fatigue depend on various factors like stress, emotional trauma, and adrenal malfunctions. Without knowing the proper cause of such symptoms, complete treatment is not possible. It is, therefore, necessary to first visit a doctor and get yourself thoroughly checked. Once the adrenal fatigue is diagnosed, there is a number of routine adjustments which are required to help adrenal glands in proper functioning. Diet in this respect is utmost important, as certain food items can cause a spark in blood pressure. To fight adrenal fatigue, the following four objectives must be kept in mind.

1. Reduced Stress Levels

2. Increased Nutrients

3. Proper adrenal function.

4. Controlled blood pressure.

What to have on an Adrenal Fatigue Diet:

A well-balanced diet is necessary to achieve most of the above-stated objectives. For an adrenal diet, certain food items are safe to have, as they don't have any impact of the blood pressure levels and adrenal glands. These are:

- whole grains
- fish
- eggs
- lean meats
- low-sugar fruits
- legumes
- leafy greens and colorful vegetables
- nuts
- dairy
- sea salt in moderation
- Good fats like olive oil, grapeseed oil, and grapeseed oil

Besides good food, hydration is also important to maintain a stable environment for the adrenal glands to work effectively. Dehydration can increase the stress levels for the body, thus taking more water and other fluids can help retain the natural balance of cortisol production.

Foods to avoid on Adrenal Fatigue Diet:

As long as we maintain the correct balance, we are allowed to enjoy most of the food items on the menu. However, there are certain elements which can aggravate the condition and should be avoided on Adrenal Fatigue diet.

- white flour
- white sugar
- caffeine
- soda
- alcohol
- processed food
- fast food
- fried food
- artificial sweeteners

It is important to note here that meal timings also hold special significance. Never skip a meal just because you are late or busy at work, especially breakfast. Take snacks in between three meals of the day and carefully maintain the balance by adding grains, vegetables, fruits, legumes and dairy products in an equal proportion. Avoid excessive salt and animal fats.

Plantain Morning Hash

Prep time: 5 minutes

Cooking time: 10 minutes

Serving: 4

Ingredients:

Hash

1 lb. breakfast sausage

3 plantains

4 tablespoons coconut oil

Chimichurri

¼ cup red wine vinegar

¼ cup balsamic vinegar

2 cloves garlic, minced

1 shallot, chopped

1 jalapeno chili, seeded, chopped

½ cup fresh basil (Thai basil)

¼ cup fresh cilantro

½ cup olive oil

1 teaspoon salt

Toppings

8 eggs, boiled

Fresh cilantro {optional}

Method:

- Blend all the ingredients for chimichurri in a food processor.
- Add plantain to a bowl and top it with chimichurri sauce.
- Slice boiled eggs and place them on the plantain.
- Garnish with cilantro.
- Serve.

Chickpea Scramble

Prep time: 10 minutes

Cooking time: 10 minutes

Serving: 2

Ingredients:

Chickpea Scramble

1 15 oz. can chickpeas

1 teaspoon turmeric

1/2 teaspoons salt

1/2 teaspoons pepper

1/4 white onion diced

2 cloves garlic minced

Olive oil, to drizzle

Breakfast Bowl

Mixed greens

A handful of parsley minced

A handful of cilantro minced

Avocado

Method:

Chickpea Scramble

- Add chickpeas to a bowl with a splash of water.
- Slightly mash them with a fork.
- Stir in salt, pepper, and turmeric. Mix well.
- Add oil to a skillet and heat over medium heat.
- Add onions and sauté for 2 to 3 minutes.
- Add garlic and saute for 30 seconds.
- Stir in chickpea mash and cook for 5 minutes with constant stirring.
- Serve the chickpea scramble with parsley, cilantro, and mixed greens.
- Garnish with avocado.
- Serve.

Apple Quinoa

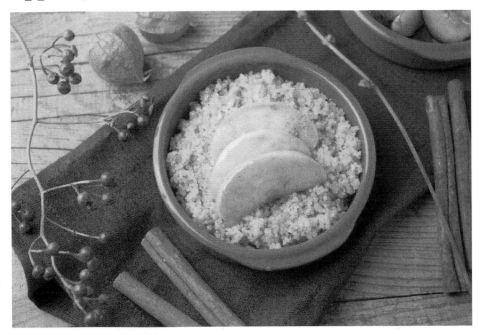

Prep time: 10 minutes

Cooking time: 35minutes

Serving: 4

Ingredients:

2 apples, grates, divided,

1 cup quinoa rinsed

1 ¼ cup almond milk

¼ cup applesauce

3 tablespoons coconut palm sugar

1 teaspoon ground cinnamon

½ teaspoon sea salt

1 teaspoon vanilla extract

Apple slices, to garnish

Method:

- Add milk and quinoa to a saucepan and bring it to a simmer.
- Stir in vanilla, applesauce, apples, salt and cinnamon.
- Let it cook for 25 minutes on low heat.
- Garnish with apple slices.
- Serve.

Sweet Potato Breakfast Bowl

Prep time: 10 minutes

Cooking time: 45 minutes

Serving: 2

Ingredients:

2 medium sweet potatoes

2/3 cup unsweetened almond milk

2 tablespoons chia seeds

1 tablespoon tahini

2 teaspoons vanilla extract

1 teaspoon cinnamon

Pinch of salt

Method:

- Spread a layer of sweet potatoes on a baking sheet.
- Bake for 45 to 60 minutes at 400 degrees F in the oven until al dente.
- Transfer the sweet potatoes flesh to a large bowl.
- Stir in all the remaining ingredients.
- Mix well using a handheld blender.

- Serve.

Egg Pancake with Kimchi

Prep time: 5 minutes

Cooking time: 5 minutes

Serving: 1

Ingredients:

1/2 tablespoon coconut oil

2-3 eggs

1/3 cup small handful kimchi

2-3 slices smoked salmon roughly chopped

1 teaspoon mayonnaise optional

1/3 cup mung bean sprouts

1/2 tablespoon sesame seeds

Chili flakes optional

Coriander, as desired

Method:

- Heat coconut oil in a frying pan.
- Whisk eggs with salt in a bowl.
- Pour this mixture into the pan and spread into a 7.8-inch circle.
- Cook for 2 minutes then flip the egg.
- Cook for another 1 to 2 minutes.
- Transfer the egg pancake to the serving plate.
- Mix kimchi with salmon and all the remaining ingredients in a bowl.

- Top the egg pancake with this mixture.
- Serve.

Shakes and Drinks

Mixed Berries Smoothie

Prep time: 10minutes

Cooking time: 10minutes

Serving: 2

Ingredients:

2 cups baby kale

1 small beet, peeled and chopped

1 cup water

1 orange, peeled

2 cups mixed berries, frozen

1 cup pineapple, frozen

1 tablespoon fresh ginger, grated or chopped

1 tablespoon coconut oil

Method:

- Add all the ingredients to a blender,
- Blend well until smooth.
- Serve.

Turmeric Latte

Prep time: 5minutes

Cooking time: 10 minutes

Serving: 1

Ingredients:

1/2 cup unsweetened almond milk

1/2 teaspoons ground turmeric

1 teaspoon ground ginger

1/2 teaspoons ground cinnamon

1/4 teaspoons ground black pepper

1 teaspoon raw honey

Method:

- Add milk, spices, and water in a saucepan.
- Cook for 10 minutes.
- Strain the mixture and allow it to cool.
- Add honey and mix well.
- Serve.

Tulsi Tea Mocktail

Prep time: 15minutes

Cooking time: 5minutes

Serving: 2

Ingredients:

2 bags of Tulsi Tea, Holy basil

16 oz. filtered water

1/4 teaspoon sea salt

2 oranges, freshly squeezed

1/2-1 tablespoon maple syrup (optional)

16 oz. of sparkling mineral water

Fresh basil leaves to taste

Method:

- Boil water in a saucepan and turn off the heat.
- Steep the tea bags in the boiled water for 4 minutes.
- Remove the tea bags then refrigerate the tea for 1 hour.
- Stir in sea salt, maple syrup, and orange juice.
- Mix well and refrigerate overnight.
- Garnish with basil leaves.
- Serve.

Cinnamon Spice Kombucha

Prep time: 10 minutes

Cooking time: 0 minutes

Serving: 1

Ingredients:

2 whole cloves

1 cinnamon stick, 3 inches long

1 teaspoon grated ginger

3 tablespoons apple juice

1¾ cup kombucha tea

Method:

- Mix apple juice with ginger and kombucha tea in a pitcher.
- Add cinnamon stick and cloves in a mason jar.
- Pour the kombucha tea into Mason jar.
- Cover the lid and allow the mixture to ferment for 5 days.
- Strain the fermented beverage through a fine sieve.
- Serve over ice cubes.

Pineapple Green Smoothie

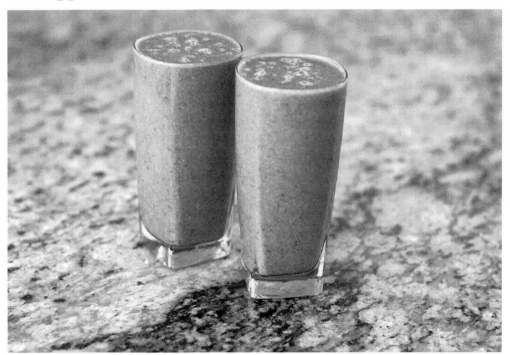

Prep time: 5minutes

Cooking time: 0 minutes

Serving: 2

Ingredients:

2 cups baby spinach

1 cup coconut water, unsweetened

1 orange, peeled

2 cups pineapple, cubed

1 cup cauliflower florets, frozen

1 teaspoon ground turmeric

2 tablespoons flax oil

Optional: adapt genic herbs

Method:

- Blend spinach with orange and coconut water in a blender until smooth.
- Add cauliflower, turmeric, pineapple, herbs and flax oil.
- Blend well again.
- Serve.

Salads

Warm Lentil and Tomato Salad

Prep time: 20 minutes

Cooking time: 50 minutes

Serving: 2

Ingredients:

Lentil Salad Dressing

1/2 cup brown lentils

10-12 sun-dried tomatoes

2-3 sprigs fresh parsley

1 tablespoon balsamic vinegar

1 teaspoon lemon juice

1 teaspoon maple syrup

1 teaspoon olive oil

1/4 teaspoons Dijon mustard

Roasted Chickpeas

1 (14oz) can chickpeas

1 teaspoon olive oil

1 teaspoon chili powder

1 pinch ground cumin

1/4 teaspoons ground turmeric

1 pinch sea salt

Method:

- Drain chickpeas and spread on a kitchen towel to absorb all the water.
- Toss chickpeas with spices and olive oil in a bowl.
- Place them on a baking sheet lined with parchment paper.
- Bake for 20 minutes at 400 degrees F in a preheated oven.
- Boil water in a saucepan and add lentils to it.
- Cook for 25 to 30 minutes.
- Drain the lentil and return it to the saucepan.
- Stir in lemon juice, olive oil, maple syrup, mustard, and vinegar.
- Mix well and let it rest 10 minutes.

- Add sliced tomatoes and parsley.
- Serve this mixture with roasted chickpeas, quinoa, and avocado slices.

Tempeh kale salad

Prep time: 5 minutes

Cooking time: 10 minutes

Serving: 4

Ingredients:

6 cups kale leaves

1 tablespoon lime juice

Tempeh

1 8 oz. block tempeh

2 tablespoons tamari

1 tablespoon lime juice

½ teaspoon onion powder

½ teaspoon cumin

¼ teaspoon chili powder

1 tablespoon olive oil

Cilantro-Lime Tahini

¼ cup cilantro leaves

3½ tablespoons water

3 tablespoons lime juice

½ teaspoon salt

5 level tbsp tahini (sesame paste)

Toppings

½ avocado, sliced

⅔ cup corn kernels

1 can black beans

1½ cup cherry tomatoes, sliced in half

Pepitas

Method:

- Toss kale leaves with 1 tablespoon lime juice in a bowl.
- Crumble the tempeh block in a medium bowl.
- Stir in lime juice and tamari. Mix well.
- Add oil to a skillet and heat over medium heat.
- Add tempeh, onion powder, chili powder, and cumin.
- Sauté for about 10 minutes until brown.
- Add all the tahini ingredients to the blender and blend until smooth.
- Mix the blended tahini dressing with the kales leaves.
- Toss in tomatoes, corn, black bean and tempeh mixture.
- Serve.

Chicken Liver Apple Salad

Prep time: 5 minutes

Cooking time: 10 minutes

Serving: 3

Ingredients:

1 cup rocket leaves

1 cup spinach leaves

½ cup blueberries

½ cup hazelnuts

1 green apple, cut into slices

1 large white onion

1 tablespoon olive oil

¾ lb. chicken livers, chopped into 1-inch pieces

The Dressing

¼ cup Lemon juice

2 tablespoons honey

2 tablespoons fresh thyme, chopped

1 clove garlic, crushed

¼ cup olive oil

Sea salt and pepper to taste

Method:

- Toss all the ingredients for salad in a bowl except livers.
- Heat 1 tablespoon oil in a skillet over medium heat.
- Add livers and sauté until golden brown.
- Transfer the cooked liver to the salad bowl.
- Combine all the ingredients of dressing in bowl.
- Pour the dressing over the salad.

- Toss well and serve.

Wakame Seaweed Salad

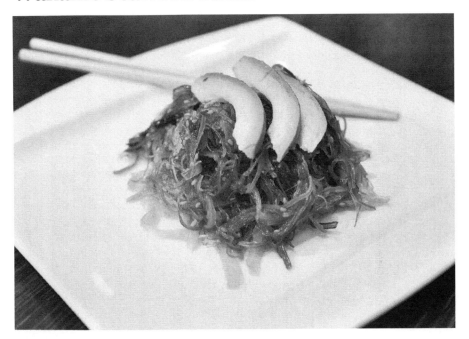

Prep time: 10 minutes

Cooking time: 10 minutes

Serving: 4

Ingredients:

2 cups baby spinach or rocket

½ cup dried wakame

1 ripe avocado

Half a cucumber

Sesame seeds

Lemon juice

Sea salt and pepper

Method:

- Soak wakame in water mixed with 2 tablespoons vinegar in a bowl for 10 minutes.
- Place the spinach leaves on the serving plate.
- Drain the wakame and transfer to a bowl.
- Toss in cucumber and avocado.
- Stir in salt, pepper, sesame seeds and lemon juice.
- Mix well and spread the mixture over the spinach.
- Garnish with avocado slices.
- Serve.

Edamame Seaweed Salad

Prep time: 10 minutes

Cooking time: 5 minutes

Serving: 4

Ingredients:

3 cups edamame

1/2 cup dried seaweed, kelp or wakame

2 green onions, sliced

1 tablespoon ginger, finely minced

2 tablespoons rice vinegar

2 tablespoons maple syrup

2 tablespoons soy sauce or tamari

1 tablespoon sesame seeds

Method:

- Boil water in a saucepan and edamame for 3 minutes.

- Drain the edamame and set them aside.
- Soak seaweed in water for 15 minutes and drain.
- Mix all the ingredients for dressing in a bow.
- Toss edamame with seaweed and dressing in a large bowl.
- Garnish with sesame seeds.
- Serve.

Main Dishes

Baked Salmon

Prep time: 5minutes

Cooking time: 20minutes

Serving: 2

Ingredients:

2 salmon filets

6 cups fresh spinach

3 large cloves of garlic, sliced

1 tablespoon parsley, finely chopped

3 teaspoon coconut oil, melted

1/4 teaspoons garlic powder

1/4 teaspoons turmeric

1/4 teaspoons turmeric

Lemon juice

Sea salt and black pepper, to taste

Method:

- Preheat your oven to 400 degrees F. Layer a baking dish with parchment paper.
- Season salmon with lemon juice, coconut oil, turmeric, garlic powder, pepper, and salt.
- Place the fish fillets in the baking dish and top them with 1 sliced garlic clove.
- Bake for about 15 minutes.
- Sauté remaining garlic in a skillet for 1 minute.
- Add spinach and cook for 2 to 3 minutes.
- Adjust seasoning with salt and pepper.
- Serve baked salmon fillets over sautéed spinach.
- Enjoy.

Bolognese Sauce with Chicken Livers

Prep time: 15minutes

Cooking time: 3hrs. 30minutes

Serving: 4

Ingredients:

2 tablespoons olive oil, divided

1 large onion, finely chopped

2 large carrots, chopped

1 large beetroot, grated

2 sticks celery, chopped

½ lb. pastured chicken livers, chopped

2 lb. grass fed beef

3 cups beef stock

3 tablespoons coconut aminos

2 bay leaves

6 stems fresh thyme

1 tablespoon fresh rosemary, chopped

1 teaspoon salt

Boiled zucchini noodles, as desired

Method:

- Preheat the oven to 250 degrees F.
- Add oil to a skillet and heat over medium heat.
- Stir in onion and sauté for 10 minutes on low heat.
- Add beetroot and carrots. Saute for 5 minutes.
- Heat remaining oil in a Dutch oven and add livers.
- Cook for 2 minutes then adds beef. Sauté for 5 minutes.
- Stir in sautéed vegetables along with herbs, coconut aminos, and stock.
- Bring it to a boil and cover the lid.
- Transfer the pan to the oven and let it cook for 3 hours.
- Remove and discard basil leaves.
- Serve with boiled zucchini noodles.

Zucchini Lasagna

Prep time: 15 minutes

Cooking time: 1 hours 15 minutes

Serving: 6

Ingredients:

Basil-Cashew Cheese

1 cup unsalted cashews, soaked and drained

½ cup unsweetened almond milk

¼ cup fresh basil leaves

2 garlic cloves

½ teaspoon sea salt

Artichoke-Tomato Sauce

1 tablespoon olive oil

1 onion, diced

2 garlic cloves, minced

14.5-ounce diced tomatoes

8-ounce tomato sauce

1 cup artichoke hearts, chopped

¼ cup fresh basil leaves, torn into pieces

Red pepper flakes, to taste

Sea salt, to taste

Freshly ground black pepper, to taste

Zucchini Lasagna

6 medium zucchinis

Coarse salt

Fresh basil, for garnish

Olive oil, for drizzling

Method:

Basil Cheese

- Blend all the ingredients in a blender.
- Serve.

Artichoke-Tomato Sauce

- Heat oil in a skillet and add onions to sauté for 3 minutes.
- Add garlic and saute for 30 seconds.
- Stir tomato sauce, tomatoes, artichoke, and basil.
- Adjust seasoning with salt, pepper, and flakes.
- Boil the mixture then reduce the heat to a simmer. Cook for 10 minutes.

Zucchini Lasagna

- Preheat your oven to 375 degrees F.
- Spread tomato sauce at the base of a casserole dish.
- Top it with a layer of zucchini slices.
- Add another layer of tomato sauce and cashew cheese.
- Repeat the layers ending with the top layer of sauce and cheese.
- Garnish with olive oil and basil.
- Cover the casserole dish and bake for 30 minutes.
- Uncover and bake for another 25 minutes.
- Allow it to rest for 15 minutes.
- Slice and serve.

Wild Rice Pilaf

Prep time: 15 minutes

Cooking time: 1hr. 5 minutes

Serving: 4

Ingredients:

1 medium butternut squash, peeled, seeded and cut into small cubes

2 cups wild rice, rinsed

6 cups vegetable stock

1 medium onion, chopped

2 cloves garlic, minced

1 cup dried cranberries

¼ cup warm water

2 tablespoons red wine vinegar

3/4 cup toasted pecans, chopped

3 tablespoons chopped Italian parsley

1/4 cup 2 tablespoons olive oil

Zest of 1 lemon

1/2 teaspoon ground cumin

1/4 teaspoon ground cardamom

1/4 teaspoon cinnamon

1/4 cup freshly squeezed lemon juice

1/4 cup freshly squeezed orange juice

1 tablespoon minced fresh ginger

Sea salt and pepper to taste

Method:

- Heat your oven to 400 degrees F.
- Toss squash pieces with salt, pepper and olive oil.
- Spread the squash on 2 baking sheets and bake for 20 minutes.
- Add oil to a skillet and heat over medium heat.

- Stir in onion and garlic and sauté for 4 minutes and set it aside.
- Soak cranberries in warm water for 10 minutes then drain.
- Mix lemon zest with olive oil, cumin, cinnamon, lemon and orange juice, cardamom and ginger in a bowl.
- Add wild rice and stock to a saucepan and cook for 40 minutes until al dente.
- Drain the rice and transfer them to a bowl.
- Toss in onions, parsley, garlic, pecans, cranberries, roasted squash, and dressing.
- Mix well and serve.

Creamy Mushroom Chicken

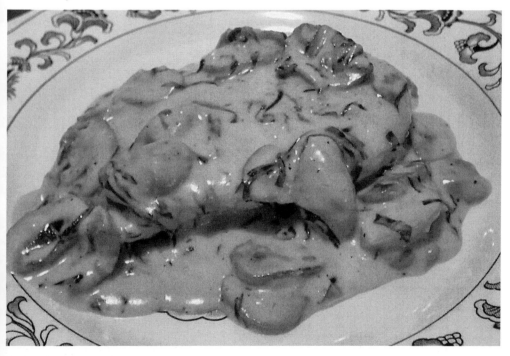

Prep time: 10 minutes

Cooking time: 15 minutes

Serving: 3

Ingredients:

3 slices bacon

6 oz. white mushrooms, sliced

2 boneless skinless chicken breasts

1 small yellow onion, chopped

1/2 red bell pepper, diced

1/2 yellow bell pepper, diced

1 tablespoon. white wine vinegar

1 14.5 oz. can coconut milk

2 cups fresh kale, stems removed & shredded

Sea salt & pepper, to taste

Method:

- Sauté bacon in a skillet until crispy.
- Transfer bacon to a plate lined with paper towel. Crumble it and set it aside.
- Add onion to the same pan and cook for 5 minutes.
- Add chicken to the pan and sear for 4 minutes per side until golden brown.
- Stir in pepper and mushrooms. Cook for 5 minutes.
- Add bacon, and white wine vinegar, coconut milk, and kale.
- Cook for 4 minutes until the sauce thickens.
- Adjust seasoning with salt and pepper.
- Serve.

Soups

Carrot and Golden Beet Soup

Prep time: 10 minutes

Cooking time: 31 minutes

Serving: 8

Ingredients:

6-7 carrots, chopped into 1/2 inch pieces

2-3 golden beets, chopped into 1/2 inch cubes

2 shallots, chopped into chunks

1 tablespoon olive oil

1/4 teaspoons ground turmeric, divided

1/4 teaspoons ground cumin, divided

1/2 teaspoons dried thyme, divided

1/2 teaspoons sea salt

2-3 cups vegetable stock

2-3 teaspoons lime juice

For serving

Chopped cilantro or parsley for serving, optional

Sliced avocado

Method:

- Layer 2 baking sheets with tin foil. Preheat the oven to 400 degrees F.
- Add carrots, beet, and shallot to the baking sheets.
- Top the veggies with spices, salt, and herbs.

- Drizzle half tbsp oil and cover the veggies with a foil sheet.
- Bake for 30minutes until al dente.
- Transfer all the ingredients to a blender.
- Puree the mixture and add the saucepan.
- Cook for 1 minute.
- Garnish with parsley and avocado.
- Serve.

Sweet Potato Green Soup

Prep time: 5 minutes

Cooking time: 25 minutes

Serving: 4

Ingredients:

2 tablespoons coconut oil

1 large onion, chopped

3 cloves garlic, minced

2-in piece ginger, peeled and minced

3 cups bone broth

1 medium white sweet potato, cubed

1 large head broccoli, chopped

1 bunch kale, chopped

1 lemon, ½ zested and juice reserved

½ teaspoon sea salt

1 bunch cilantro

Avocado for garnish

Method:

- Add and heat oil in a skillet. Stir in onions.
- Sauté for 7 minutes then add ginger and garlic. Cook for 1 minute.
- Stir in sweet potato, broccoli, and broth.
- Boil the soup then reduce the heat to a simmer.
- Cook for 15 minutes then turn off the heat.
- Add all the remaining ingredients.
- Puree the mixture using a handheld blender.
- Garnish with cilantro and avocado.
- Serve warm.

Lentil Spinach Soup

Prep time: 10minutes

Cooking time: 10 minutes

Serving: 4

Ingredients:

1/2 onion

2 carrots

1 rib celery

1 clove garlic

2 tablespoons tomato paste

1 teaspoon dried vegetable broth powder

1 teaspoon Sazon seasoning

1 cup red lentils

1 tablespoon lemon juice

3 cups filtered water

1 bunch spinach

Method:

- Heat oil in a pot and add all the vegetables.
- Sauté for 5 minutes then add broth, tomato paste, and Sazon seasoning.
- Mix well and stir in red lentils along with water.
- Cook until lentil is soft and tender.
- Add spinach and cook for 2 minutes.
- Serve warm with lemon slices on top.

Tangy Lentil Soup

Prep time: 15minutes

Cooking time: 20minutes

Serving: 4

Ingredients:

2 cups red lentils, picked over and rinsed

1 serrano chile pepper, chopped

1 large tomato, roughly chopped

1 1 1/2-inch piece ginger, peeled and grated

3 cloves garlic, finely chopped

1/4 teaspoon ground turmeric

Sea salt, to taste

Topping

Fresh cilantro, chopped, for topping

1/4 cup Greek yogurt

Method:

- Add lentils to a pot and with enough water to cover it.
- Bring the lentils to a boil then reduce the heat.
- Cook for 10 minutes on low simmer.
- Stir in all the remaining ingredients.
- Cook until lentils are soft and well mixed.
- Garnish with fresh cilantro and dollop of yogurt.
- Serve.

Broccoli Cheese Soup

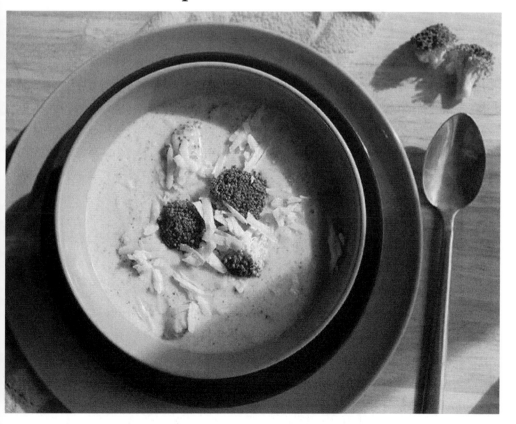

Prep time: 10minutes

Cooking time: 40 minutes

Serving: 10

Ingredients:

4 heads broccoli, cut into 1-inch pieces

Olive oil, for drizzling

Sea salt and freshly ground black pepper

4 ounces unsalted butter

1 whole onion, diced

1/3 cup all-purpose flour

4 cups whole milk

2 cups half-and-half cream

Pinch nutmeg

3 cups grated cheddar cheese

1 cup chicken broth, optional

Method:

- Toss broccoli florets with oil, and pepper.
- Spread the florets on a baking sheet.
- Bake at 375 degrees F in a preheated oven until crispy.
- Heat butter in a pot and add onions.
- Sauté for 4 minutes then sprinkle flour on it.
- Mix well and cook for 1 minute.
- Stir in half and half cream and milk.
- Add roasted broccoli, nutmeg, salt, and pepper.
- Cover the pot and cook for 30 minutes on low heat.

- Add cheese and allow it to melt in.
- Lightly blend the soup using a handheld blender.
- Garnish with shredded cheese and broccoli florets.
- Serve warm.

Snacks

Kale Chips

Prep time: 10 minutes

Cooking time: 12 minutes

Serving: 6

Ingredients:

1 bunch kale, leaves only

1 tablespoon olive oil

1 teaspoon seasoned salt

Method:

- Set the oven to 350 degrees F. Layer a cookie sheet with parchment paper.
- Tear the kale leaves in small pieces and toss them with oil and salt.
- Spread them on the prepared cookie sheet.
- Bake for 12 minutes.
- Serve.

Goji Berry Nut Bars

Prep time: 10minutes

Cooking time: 25 minutes

Serving: 12

Ingredients:

1 cup raw almonds

½ cup pistachios

½ cup desiccated coconut, unsweetened

½ cup pumpkin seeds

½ cup sunflower seeds

4 tablespoons chia seeds

2 tablespoons lemon zest

1 teaspoon vanilla bean extract

½ cup goji berries

½ teaspoon cinnamon

3 tablespoons coconut oil, melted

½ cup honey

Method:

- Layer a 9 inch baking pan with parchment paper.
- Preheat the oven to 350 degrees F.
- Mix all the ingredients except nut in a bowl until fluffy.
- Fold in chopped nuts.
- Pour the nutty batter into the baking pan and press firmly.
- Bake for 25 minutes until golden brown.
- Allow it to cool then chop into smaller pieces.
- Serve.

Wasabi Deviled Eggs

Prep time: 10 minutes

Cooking time: 10 minutes

Serving: 8

Ingredients:

8 eggs

½ teaspoon rice vinegar

½ teaspoon wasabi

½ teaspoon crushed ginger

½ sheet nori, chopped into 1/2 cm pieces

2 tablespoons yogurt

Spring onions, finely chopped

Mild chili powder

Method:

- Boil water in a pot and add eggs to cook.
- Cook for 10 minutes then drain and rinse them under cold water.
- Peel eggs and slice them in two halves.
- Remove yolks from the middle of each egg and transfer them to a bowl.
- Add nori, yogurt, rice vinegar, ginger and wasabi to the yolks.
- Mix and mash well using a fork.
- Transfer this yolk mixture into a piping bag with a star-shaped tip.
- Pipe mashed yolk into the center all the egg whites.
- Garnish with spring onions and chili powder.
- Serve.

Zucchini Chips

Prep time: 10minutes

Cooking time: 10 minutes

Serving: 2

Ingredients:

2 zucchini

2 tablespoons olive oil

Sea salt

Method:

- Heat your oven to 250 degrees F.
- Thinly slice the zucchini and spread the slices on a kitchen towel.
- Sprinkle salt on the slice and let them rest for 10 minutes.
- Toss the dried zucchini slices with oil and spread them on 2 baking sheets.
- Bake for 1 hour until crispy.
- Serve with your favorite dip.

Cinnamon Sweet Potato Chips

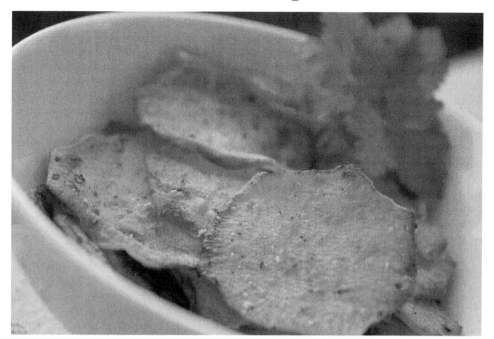

Prep time: 15minutes

Cooking time: 20minutes

Serving: 4

Ingredients:

2 sweet potatoes, peeled and thinly sliced

1 tablespoon melted butter

1/2 teaspoon salt

2 teaspoons brown sugar

1/2 teaspoon ground cinnamon

Method:

- Grease 2 cookie sheets. Preheat the oven to 400 degrees F.
- Toss the sweet potato slices with salt, butter, cinnamon and brown sugar.

- Spread these slices in the baking sheets.
- Bake for 23 minutes until crispy.
- Serve.

Desserts

Vanilla Ice Cream

Prep time: 5minutes

Cooking time: 0 minutes

Serving: 4

Ingredients:

2 cups water

1 cup raw cashews

1/4 cup raw honey

1 tablespoon vanilla extract

Sea salt (to taste)

Method:

- Add all the ingredients to a blender
- Blend well until smooth.
- Pour this mixture into the ice cream makes.
- Churn the ice cream as per the given instructions of the ice cream maker.
- Serve.

Cocoa Mousse

Prep time: 5minutes

Cooking time: 0minutes

Serving: 2

Ingredients:

2 ripe avocados

3 tablespoons full fat coconut milk

1/4 cup unsweetened cocoa powder

2 tablespoons raw honey

1 teaspoon vanilla extract

Sea salt, to taste

Chopped almonds, walnuts or coconut flakes

Fresh cilantro

Method:

- Blend avocado flesh with cocoa powder, honey, coconut milk, salt and vanilla extract in a blender.
- Pour in more coconut milk if the mixture is too thick.
- Garnish with walnuts, almonds and coconut flakes.
- Serve.

Coconut Flour Brownies

Prep time: 10 minutes

Cooking time: 40 minutes

Serving: 8

Ingredients:

¾ cup coconut flour

¼ cup almond flour

1 cup cocoa powder

1 cup coconut oil, melted

¾ cup honey

6 eggs

1 teaspoon vanilla bean paste

Method:

- Grease a 9-inch brownie pan and preheat the oven to 320 degrees F.
- Combine all dry ingredients to a bowl.
- Whisk honey with eggs, coconut oil, and vanilla bean paste.
- Stir in dry mixture and mix well until smooth.
- Pour the batter into the greased pan.
- Bake for 30 to 40 minutes.
- Serve.

Rice Custard

Prep time: 15 minutes

Cooking time: 2 hr. 30 minutes

Serving: 2

Ingredients:

4 cups milk

1/2 cup sugar

1/4 cup rice, uncooked

Zest from 1 lemon

1/4 teaspoons salt

2 eggs, well beaten

1/2 cup raisins

Cinnamon to taste

Method

- Preheat the oven to 325 degrees F.
- Mix milk with lemon peel, salt, rice and sugar in a bowl.
- Pour this mixture in a 2-quart casserole dish.
- Place the casserole dish into a baking pan filled with water up to 1 inch.
- Bake for 1 hour in the oven.
- Remove the dish from the oven and give a gentle stir.
- Bake again for 45 minutes.
- Beat this hot milk mixture with eggs and return it to the casserole dish.
- Fold in raisins and bake for another 30 minutes.
- Garnish with cinnamon.
- Serve warm.

Chocolate Cake

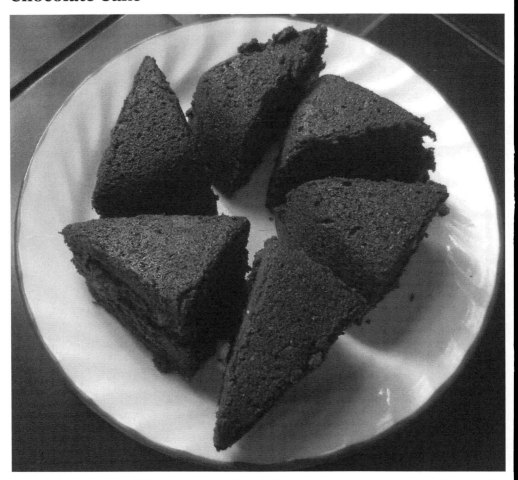

Prep time: 15 minutes

Cooking time: 30 minutes

Serving: 6

Ingredients:

3 1/2 oz. of sweet chocolate

1/2 cup boiling water

6 eggs, separated

2 cups sugar, divided

1 cup butter

1 teaspoon pure vanilla extract

2 cups rice flour

2 tablespoons cornstarch

1 teaspoon baking powder

1 teaspoon baking soda

1/2 teaspoons salt

1 cup buttermilk

Method:

- Preheat your oven to 350 degrees F.
- Boil water in a pot and top it with a glass bowl.
- Add chocolate in the bowl and cook until it melts.
- Beat egg whites in an electric mixer until foamy.
- Whisk in half cup sugar and beat again until smooth.
- Beat butter with remaining sugar and vanilla until fluffy.
- Stir in egg yolks and melted chocolate.
- Blend well and set it aside.
- Mix flour with baking powder, salt, baking soda and cornstarch in a bowl.
- Gradually add the dry mixture into the yolks mixture.
- Fold in egg whites and mix gently.
- Pour the batter into the baking pan and bake for 30 minutes at 350 degrees F.
- Serve.

Conclusion:

Adrenal fatigue is natural to the ongoing living changes, inactive lifestyle and unhealthy dietary habits. With minute adjustments in the routine meal and little care, we can to avoid the exhaustive symptoms of Adrenal Fatigue. Treatment through better food and exercise is proved to be far more effective than any other medical methods. It is safe and long lasting. This book is therefore designed to focus on the hormonal deficiencies due to adrenal malfunction and its impact on the body, while bringing out the best possible solution through a complete and consolidated Adrenal Fatigue diet plan. All the recipes are divided into different sections to cater to everyone's daily needs, from breakfast to beverage, salads, main meals, soups, snacks, and desserts. Using these recipes anyone can create a combination which could suit their caloric intake and personal taste preferences.

Printed in Great Britain
by Amazon

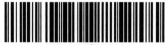
44266477R00029